The Ancient Science of Reflexology: A Beginner's Guide to Reducing Stress, Toxins, and Improving Health

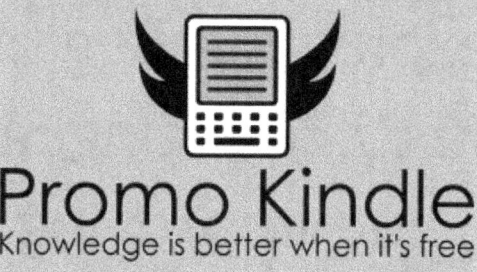

Disclaimer

"The Ancient Science of Reflexology: A Beginner's Guide to Reducing Stress, Toxins, and Improving Health"

Copyright © 2015 – All Rights Reserved

The information included in this book is for educational purposes only and is not meant to be a substitute for seeking the advice of a professional. The author and publisher have made their best efforts to ensure that the information in this book is accurate. However, they make no warranties as to the accuracy or completeness of the contents herein and cannot be held responsible for any errors, omissions, or dated material. This book contains methods and other advice that, regardless of my own results and experience, may not produce the same results (or any results) for you. The author makes absolutely no guarantee, expressed or implied, that by following the advice, or using the data below readers can get the same results, as there are several factors and variables that come into play regarding any given situation.

Liability Disclaimer:

What This Book Has For You

Just like many other alternative healing therapies, reflexology therapy was also viewed with skepticism for a very long time. However, it amazed people with how it actually works – and if you are looking for answers and solutions, this book will be your guide about how it exactly works and why is this alternative therapy one of the most effective ones practiced to date.

The practice of applying pressure to specific points on the hands and feet to relieve stress and to influence health is what reflexology is all about. This simple act can actually make your life better and stress free if you know how to do it. This comprehensive yet approachable guide explains how reflexology works – simply by applying pressure to 'reflex' points on your feet and hands. This helps stimulate the natural powers of the body to begin self-healing.

This book covers the following topics in detail for your better understanding of the ancient practice:

1. Introduction to reflexology and how it works.
2. History of reflexology to help you understand where it all started and how it became popular as one of the most effective alternative therapies for self-healing.
3. The overall benefits of reflexology and its impact on your lifestyle.
4. The book also reveals myths that are associated with this ancient practice.
5. A detailed reflexology chart that explains the internal system of your hands and feet, pressure points, and how to use reflexology successfully.
6. Techniques that can be used to de-stress your body using reflexology.
7. Tips and tricks used to remove toxins from your body with the help of reflexology practices.

8. Tips and tricks to make the most out of reflexology techniques to gain maximum benefits for your body.
9. How to self-practice reflexology on your own hands and feet for benefits.
10. The book also contains amazing DIY techniques that can be incorporated into your daily lives and busy schedules.

With all that information in hand, you will definitely be in a better position to use the magical, relaxing techniques to achieve great results. This book features fully illustrated sequences of reflexology for different scenarios and for all ages, this relaxing, calming technique will help you forge better relationships and stronger bonds with people in your life, and bring a gentle healing touch in your personality.
So read the book till the end and use the information in your best interest.
Get started now, good luck!

Contents

Introduction to Reflexology

They say… you can change your life with the techniques of reflexology. This claim conjures up all the possibilities associated with the benefits of reflexology. It implies at the potential of having a positive impact on the overall quality of life, as well as your health. The phrase also suggests that with the help of reflexology, one can gain innumerable amount of benefits starting from the earliest infancy days to the golden years.

Have you ever tried using reflexology for improving your health? It is important to understand that reflexology cannot be simply regarded as just theoretical exercise. For us, as well as for millions of others who have been using this technique throughout history, the alternative healing practice of reflexology helps with self-healing and gives the sense of being able to do anything in the world.

There's no rocket science attached to it. In fact, the magic lies within your own fingertips. It is your own ability that you can use whenever you want. The technique empowers you to accept the different stages of life and address all the challenges positively.

This book speaks to the application of reflexology at different points in our lives. In fact, if you think about it, you will realize that reflexology has been there around us all the while to cope and calm us.

Whether it is to ease down the pre-wedding jitters of the bride to post-wedding tired feet, to heal someone's sports injury or to calm pregnancy troubles, reflexology has helped us smoothed the way. The ability to utilize this practice has helped us all in challenging times.

Reflexology can help a 97-year old to fight distress just as effectively as it would to an infant. It is a great way to address allergies, constipation, kidney stones, menstruation, colic, pregnancy, heart problems, flesh-eating bacteria, accident injury, foot and back problems, swollen ankles… and we could go on and on.

As you start using this technique on yourself, you will find that one success leads to another, and this chain process goes on.

The History of Reflexology – How It All Started

The history of Reflexology –as per the evident –traces back to the ancient Egypt. The origin of this technique was evidenced by inscriptions found on the tomb of a physician at Saqqara in Egypt. The hieroglyphics on the tomb had the following message in translation: "Don't hurt me." The practitioner's reply: "I shall act so you praise me."

Although we cannot exactly determine the type of relationship between the ancient Egypt art as practiced by the natives and reflexology, it definitely had its roots belonging there. In fact, different forms of feet work have been practiced all over the ancient world for health.

The theory of 'Zone' was the originator of modern techniques of Reflexology, which all started with Dr. William H. Fitzgerald, M.D. whom Dr. Edwin Bowers, M.D., motivated to publish all the articles he had written on the unique subject of 'Zone Analgesia'. Later in 1917, both Dr. William and Dr. Edwin published a book called 'Relieving Pain At Home'. In the book they mentioned, "Humanity is awakening to the fact that sickness, in a large percentage of cases, is an error – of body and mind." Eventually, people start believing it and soon it became a universal truth. Dr. William H. Fitzgerald was a specialist of throat, nose and ear working actively as a doctor at the St. Francis Hospital as well as Boston City Hospital in Connecticut.

He named his work 'Zone Analgesia' in which pressure was applied to zones or the bony eminence corresponding to the area of pain or injury. He also introduced using pressure points at the back of the pharynx, on the palate, and tongue in order to achieve positive result of analgesia or pain relief. He did this by utilizing a number of tools including aluminum combs, clothes pegs, and elastic bands, for the hands, regular palpebral retractor and nasal probes for the pharynx, and surgical clamps to be used on the tongue. Dr. William was the first person responsible for coming up with the first charge about the longitudinal zones of the body.

Another very interesting discovery of Dr. Fitzgerald was the application of pressure on the injured or painful zones did not only help in relieving pain but in most of the cases also helped in controlling or reliving the underlying cause.

This is exactly what we can achieve from reflexology today. It is believed that the technique is based partially on Dr. William's Zone Theory. Dr. Fitzgerald together with Dr. Shelby Riley further worked on the theory and developed it further. Horizontal zones were added to the longitudinal zones of the body across the hands and feet. This helped them determine individual reflexes according to the Zone Theory. Another Physical Therapist, Eunice D. Ingham, joined hands with Dr. Riley out of the fascination she had with the Zone Therapy. Following the same techniques, she developed her foot reflex theory and introduced it during the 1930s. She treated hundreds of patients using this technique considering each reflex point as a mirror image of the body organs. Each reflex point was checked thoroughly until she was confident to use the reflexes on the feet to achieve results.

She found inspiration to write from Dr. Riley and published her first book "Stories The Feet Can Tell" in 1938. In this book, she documented the cases she handled and mapped out the possible reflexes that looked like body organs on the feet –we know them as reflexology today.

The first book by Eunice D Ingham was later translated into multiple foreign languages that spread the word about the benefits one can achieve using Reflexology techniques. The translated versions of the book in seven different languages helped people benefit beyond the border of United States.

It was at this point that the confusion between Zone Therapy and Reflexology started. This happened because some foreign publishers named Eunice's book as 'Zone Therapy' and unfortunately, in some parts of the world people still think that Zone Therapy and Reflexology are same techniques. However, both these therapies are different from each other by a distinct feature. While Zone Therapy totally relies on the zones to determine the affected area to be worked on, Reflexology focuses on both the zones as well as the anatomical model.

After the publication and popularity of her book, Eunice D Ingham traveled around the country to hold different health workshops and for book reviews. Dilapidated and sick people attended these workshops and book review programs where she would share her knowledge with the people by discussing and working on different health problems they have been facing.

During the late 50s, Dwight Byers started to work closely with Eunice Ingham and helped her with her programs and workshops. Later in the year 1961, Dwight Byers along with his sister Eusebia Messenger joined the workshops of Aunt Eunice. After seven years, both the siblings were responsible to continue the teachings of Reflexology under 'The National Institute of Reflexology' banner. Eusebia retired during the mid-70s and Dwight Byers continued and formed 'The International Institute of Reflexology', where he further put in his efforts to refine the techniques and understandings of Reflexology.

Eunice D. Ingham died at the age of 85 in the year 1974. However, her teachings that Reflexology can aid in easing down the sufferings continued to prosper and spread across the world. The undisputable contributions of Eunice Ingham of Reflexology that she shared with the world included the following:

1. She discovered that reflexes on a human's feet are exactly like the organs inside the body. She charted the map of reflexes in the same manner as the anatomical model for easier identification.
2. She further stressed on the understanding that alternating pressure can add a stimulating effect on the body instead of numbing the affected area. This was also demonstrated by Dr. William Fitzgerald.
3. She did not only introduce Reflexology to the non-medical community and general public, but also to Physiotherapists, Massage Therapist, Osteopaths, Chiropodists, and Naturopaths.

After the death of Eunice D. Ingham, Dwight Byres along with his wife Nancy continued to consolidate and formulate the teachings of Aunt Eunice through the International Institute of Reflexology that he launched. He later on wrote a number of books to further stress down on the teachings of Reflexology. He showed sincere dedication towards his Aunt Eunice by promoting the techniques of Reflexology as a healthier way of achieving great health. He promoted Reflexology in the United States and a number of other countries including New Zealand, Australia, South America, South Africa, Israel, Europe, and Singapore.

These are some important names in the history who have developed, pioneered and build the strong foundation of Reflexology as we know it today.

Understanding the Science of Reflexology

The technique of reflexology requires skills that are based on scientific foundations. It is a great, gentle art that is fascinated by ancient science. Reflexology is a highly effective type of therapeutic foot and hand massage that does not only have an interesting history but have also made into the field of complementary medicine in today's modern world. The technique is based on both art and science, art because a significant part of the technique depends on how skillfully the knowledge is gained and applied by the therapist and science because the technique of reflexology is based on neurological and physiological study.

Referring back to the history, it was discovered that feet are a microcosm of a human body. All the body parts, glands and organs are represented as a mirror image on the feet.

The science behind the technique also suggests that reflexology works on the premise that the organs we have in our body have reflexes on our feet and by stimulating those reflexes, one can actually stimulate the different body parts and encourage the body to heal naturally.

Reflexology maps the entire according to the internal structure of our body. The map includes the toes and the entire feet to represent our body organs. Expert finger and thumb techniques are use to apply pressure on the reflexes to heal and calm body. The stimulation caused by the pressure brings physiological changes to take place in the body and boosts the healing potential.

For general understanding, the science behind the Reflexology technique states that when the reflex area has some sensitivity, it is an indication of weakness or stress in the corresponding body part or organ.

Following the same science, it is believed that reflexology helps in restoring balance in the body, boosting its healing power by inducing relaxation. By applying pressure on the sensitive parts, the homeostasis is triggered that brings back balance or the state of equilibrium in the body.

The best way to achieve this balance is by inducing relaxation and reducing stress or tension from your body. It is also important to understand that when the body is relaxed, it is in the best state for effective healing.

In short, reflexology is a holistic approach of treatment that incorporates body, spirit and mind.

Reflexology aims to heal the body by treating it from deep down the root cause of the problem or disease. So when you turn to reflexology for body healing, know that you will be treating much more than just symptoms. For desirable results, it is important that the patient also participate actively when the therapy is going on. In all types of holistic therapies, it is very important for the patient to be active and take responsibility for one's own health.

How Reflexology Works

As mentioned earlier, reflexologists use their fingers and thumb to apply pressure techniques to the feet and hands to stimulate certain reflex areas in order to produce a beneficial response to the corresponding organ or part of the body. Reflexologists often refer to the map (covered later in the book) to correspond different reflex areas to the different body parts, glands and organs inside the body. This helps them create a mirror image of the body in the feet as well as the hands and helps the self-help practitioners as well as professional reflexologists to easily target the affected area on the hand or foot to work on.

When there is danger in the environment close to our body, it actives the survival mechanism known as the 'fight or flight'. When the body is responding to the exposed danger, it gathers information from the environment and instantly transfers it to the brain, muscles, and internal organs in order to prepare them for taking appropriate action. Both hands and feet actively participate in this response.

Responsive Feet

"The feet act as self-tuners for the rest of the body: movements of the feet is important for the stimulation of the whole system"

During the survival mechanism, the feet are highly responsive and prepared to participate in fleeing or defending. This happens by processing the information gather from the environment through pressure sensors present in the soles. The process helps body determine optimum oxygen and fuel levels.

For instance, you need more oxygen for running than simply walking. Similarly, feet that need to take off require different ranges of oxygen and fuel than what it needs to prepare to fight or to stand firm.

In order to achieve the right balance of oxygen and fuel, pressure signals collected by the soles inform the brain whether the body is lying down, sitting or standing. This enables the feel to decide whether muscle relaxation and contraction, oxygen and blood sugar needs are currently at the required level. In case it is not, the brain sends signals to the body to make the required adjustments accordingly.

Now think about a situation when someone is running or jogging. Do you know what it takes for the body to prepare for it? Since running or jogging requires increased pressure to the feet, the message is sent to the brain that the person is running and adjustments are made accordingly.

The brain tells the body to adjust the organs in a way that helps the body produce more energy to keep up with jogging. With time, your body becomes conditioned to jog better as you continue to produce more energy and build stamina. Reflexology is jogging without any weight since the technique requires application of similar pressure without the demands of weight-bearing or standing. For instance, one major nerve connects the brain with the center of the big toe. The same nerve is responsible for controlling cardiac acceleration, respiration, and movement. Therefore, when pressure is applied to this area, a revival response is triggered by the pituitary gland reflex area.

Responsive Hands

Hands help us to survive. We use them to reach out to the whole world, defending and befriending as well as working and picking up the pieces when required.

Our hands are also blessed with natural pressure sensors that helps us to communicate with people around us and allow us to manipulate our surroundings, perform routinely tasks, carry out daily household and office-related chores, and use different tools that makes our lives easier.

Just like our feet – at the fundamental point – are essential for our survival, taking care of ourselves and our hygiene, nurturing the young ones, providing food, creating shelter – what not! And most importantly, when our body is exposed to danger, our hands also participate in the same survival mechanism – 'Fight or Flight Response' – like our feet.

The sudden urge to lift up your little one when he/she is exposed to some danger is the best example of an extraordinary response of your hands.

Interrupted Patterns of Stress

Similar stress mechanism is active when we are regularly responding to the daily demands of the day. While we are actively participating and keeping up with those demands, doing so on a continuous basis leaves our body in a wear and tear condition.

According to Hans Selye (1907 – 1982) – a researcher – more than 75% of illnesses are a result of stress. He further convinced that the pattern of stress provides a break in the routine, which helps us improve our condition and get rid of the continuous stress.

Foot and hand reflexology works in this situation by interrupting stress and resets the overall level of tension in the body. As our feet and hands actively respond to these sensory experiences of pressure techniques of reflexology, it interrupts the stress pattern and instantly give your body great feeling of relaxation.

The Benefits of Reflexology

Some of the most common benefits of reflexology include its ability to increase energy, induce great levels of relaxation, stimulate nerve function, boost circulation, stimulate central nervous system, remove toxins from the body, cleans up urinary tract conditions, prevents migraines, helps relieve sleep disorders, reduces depression, speeds up recovery after surgery or injury, and relieves pain.

Moreover, it is a great natural technique and to ease different ailments.

Reflexology is a great holistic approach with great benefits for all ages. It can relieve you from a long list of chronic and acute conditions. In addition to the benefits mentioned above, reflexology is a technique also considered effective for:

a. Menopause
b. Headaches and migraines
c. Hormonal imbalances
d. Back pain
e. Circulatory problems
f. Sleeping disorders
g. Arthritis
h. Stress related disorders
i. Digestive problems
j. Allergies
k. Insomnia
l. Blood pressure
m. Asthma
n. Constipation
o. Eczema
p. Bowel disorder
q. Frozen shoulder
r. Hay fever
s. Knee problems

t. *Multiple sclerosis*
u. *Neck problems*
v. *Muscle tension*
w. *Sinusitis*
x. *Thyroid imbalance*
y. *Respiratory problems*
z. *Gynecological disorders*

Here are the Benefits in Detail:

a. *Stress Relief* – One of the main reasons why people turn to reflexology is to get relief from stress. Whether you suffer from fatigue, digestive problems, migraines or insomnia, the root of most of these health issues could be associated with stress. Stress is usually a cause of environmental, physical, and emotional factors around us as well as our hectic lifestyle. In short, in most cases, avoiding stress can be totally impossible. The sad part is that this unavoidable situation can be damaging to our mind and body. Under the influence of prolonged and high levels of stress, our body becomes more prone to developing illnesses. Since reflexology is a technique that is known for promoting relaxation and bringing a natural balance to our system, it can effectively counteract the unwanted effects of stress.

b. *Improved Circulation* – Our system require proper blood circulation to function effectively. Proper blood circulation ensures oxygen and nutrients are carried throughout the body via cells while ridding the body of toxins and waste products. Tension and stress can mess with our cardiovascular system and restrict blood flow. This could make our system sluggish. Eventually, the cells and tissues in our body are deprived of oxygen and our body becomes depleted. The techniques of reflexology keep the circulation of blood in the body smooth, which rejuvenates cells and tissues.

c. *Muscle Relaxation* – There are a number of factors that could lead to muscle tension, for instance, keeping your body in one position for a very long time, working out using heavy weights, lifting heavy objects, or emotional stress. Regardless of your individual situation, when muscles are tense, energy is stressed and our system falls out of balance. It further congests our nerve pathway that connects our body through different muscles. This may lead to further stress, irritability, fatigue, and even excruciating pain. When the techniques of reflexology are applied, it effectively stimulates nerve endings and releases energy in the body. Reflexology not only restores physical harmony but also relaxes muscles.

d. *Cleanse and Detoxify* – It is extremely important for our body to get rid of toxins and waste. When the intestinal, urinary, or lymphatic systems are blocked because of waste products and toxins, it makes the body stagnate. This further leads to making you feel sicker, lethargic, and bloated. Reflexology can help you deal with these blockages. When the blockage is released, it helps your body to eliminate waste products and toxins in the body. Reflexology is a great technique to cleanse your system from all sorts of impurities. This further helps the body to retain balance and restore itself naturally.

e. *Headaches and Migraines* – Since reflexology is a very common technique practiced for eliminating pain, people turn to this to ease down headaches and severe migraines. As an analgesic treatment, reflexology can effectively help you reduce severity of headaches and migraines by relieving the associated muscles from tension. It is also effective in eliminating headaches that are induced by stress, since psychological and stress factors often show up through physical symptoms. In fact, treating migraines and headaches are two of the most popular applications of this holistic technique.

f. *Speeds the Process of Healing* – Reflexology has great benefits in improving blood circulation and nerve activity. This combination along with more effective metabolism indicates growth of cells at a much faster pace. This is what helps wounds to heal faster. In addition to this, the pain-relieving characteristics of reflexology are very positive for patients who want to feel better and restart their life quickly after physical recovery.

g. *Body Balancer* – To maintain the right balance is healthy for our body, spirit, and mind. The body must function properly in order to maintain the right state of homeostasis. When your body experiences malfunction, it comes out of the natural balance automatically. Reflexology is essential for sustaining balance in every cell, tissue, muscle, organ, and gland present in the body, and setting it back to the natural balance.

Is Reflexology Beneficial For me?

By using your hands and feet for pressure application on different reflex points, the lymph flow and blood circulation of the body improves. This helps your system to get rid of toxins and impurities present in your body and revitalizes energy. This further encourages the body to naturally restore its own healthy balance.

In addition to this, reflexology can help bring relaxation and soothing to your body, spirit, and mind. In short, the treatment is highly beneficial for anyone who believes in it and pursues it as a method of healing and natural treatment. By opting for reflexology, you will undergo a treatment that is extremely relaxing and pleasurable to receive, as well as energizing and invigorating.

Building Physical Awareness

We are on our feet most of the times during the day. We use our hands to carry out different tasks throughout the day until we finally go to sleep. The repetitive nature of routine life causes wear and tear on our feet and hands, and minimizes their natural capabilities.

Keeping up with the daily dose of life, our hands and feet not only become tired but also experience limitation in their function. The technique of reflexology for creating physical awareness hides in offering the right exercise treatment to our feet and hands to bring them back to their full natural capabilities. These vital parts of our body are effective sensory organs and introducing them to variety will only help them contribute at their best to achieve great living and healthy development.

One of the most common complaints of people who visit reflexologists is that they feel constant pain in their feet. Once they are done with the reflexology session, they have exactly the opposite comment. They feel relaxed and soft and feel as if they are walking on soft cotton pillows. This response is a result of the unaccustomed sensation they experience in their feet, which is a result of pressure techniques followed in reflexology. The variation of pressures from hard underfoot surfaces during the session calms down nerves, relaxes the person, and relieves pain.

The same is with the hands. Since the hands also experience the same level (or more for some people) of repetitive activities during the day, getting a reflexology session for your hands will also give you the same level of satisfaction.

Education for Feet and Hands

The best part about using reflexology as an alternative treatment is that the benefits offered by this technique are not temporary or short term. In fact, education is provided to the feet and hands during the session as to how they should feel at best. It is very important to provide awareness, as this is an aid for using your most vital body parts more effectively. For instance, a person who underwent the reflexology therapy and learned self-help relaxing technique gained immense benefits to ease down the feet pain he gained by standing in the classroom for years. The pain became so severe with time that he reached a point where his career as a teacher was at risk.

However, once he got familiar with the right method to take care of his feet, he was in a better position to counteract the effects and pain of long hours of standing.

Ever seen new moms giving their newborns a soft massage on their hands and feet? Ever noticed how they used their fingers and thumbs to apply pressure on the reflex points? Educated moms often do this to provide the right level of stimulation that the hands and feet receive as they know the fundamental role it plays in the development of their babies.

Children as they grow up learn the most basics of skills through reflexology and surprise us by climbing stairs or using their hands to pick up things from the floor. This is because their brain practiced initiating motion for lifting themselves and other objects through the basic skill of reflexology.

In short, the physical education they receive in the form of reflexology as newborn babies does not end there. In fact, they adapted those positive changes and constantly developed with their changing environment as they grew up. They constantly used their sensory body parts to gain education and apply the information.

The awareness or education that the hands and feet gained during the early stage of life can serve a human being for a lifetime. Just like using good toothpaste and brushing can preserve our teeth, similarly, by stimulating hands and feet through regular reflexology can work out as precaution against losing physical functions in later life.

On the other hand, educating your feet and hands and giving them physical awareness will help you maintain independent style of living. Reflexology is beneficial for younger people as well as for the older generation. While learning the basic skills at a young age will help you carry on effectively for the rest of your life, for elderly people it teaches them the right way to retain their mobility by making the most out of their legs, feet and walking habits and the right way of using their hands. This further reduces the risk of developing a number of health problems.

The Myths of Reflexology

Since reflexology is a popular technique, there are always people who try to defame it. People who spread the wrong word about reflexology also include those who failed to benefit from the technique because of their wrong approach. Unfortunately, people pick up these myths much faster than they would the benefits.

So before we proceed, here are some common myths of reflexology that you should not believe.

1. **Reflexology is a very painful procedure. Unless you really feel the pain, it will not be effective.** This is a very common thing you will hear from a lot of people. Unfortunately, these statements also come from people who have experienced it. The truth is that reflexology is not painful. In fact, the way the pressure is applied to hands and feet is actually relaxing. It is more like getting a full body massage after working for a month. The calming and soothing properties of reflexology are what make it one of the most desirable alternative treatments people look for these days.

2. **The techniques used in reflexology are all same. In case you find if one practitioner is different from the other, one of them is doing is wrong.** You will get a clearer idea about the reality here when you will go through the nest chapter about Reflexology Maps. For now, know that there are different techniques used for applying pressure to address the different problems you are facing. If one practitioner is doing it differently from the other one, it does not indicate anything wrong. In fact, they both might be addressing your issues in different ways.

3. **They use needles in reflexology.** This is where they confuse reflexology with acupuncture. Needles are used in acupuncture and not reflexology. So if you are scared of the needles or not ready to take the pain of those pricks, you can still go for reflexology for your relaxation without any fear.

4. **Reflexology is some sort of spiritual stuff or maybe black magic.** Seriously? Well, this is one of the myths that sound extremely idiotic. It's simply a procedure of massaging your hand and feet and activating the sensory characteristics of your vital organs for great benefits. The process is naturally, beneficial for health, and spiritually healing. There's nothing related to black magic or spiritual stuff associated with reflexology.

5. **Reflexology is nothing but just a type of massages that offers temporary pleasure and stress relief.** That's another big misconception about reflexology. In fact, the benefits are permanent and set up as your basic, fundamental skills that you learn at tender age and offers you benefits even when you get old. The benefits you gain from this technique are permanent and lifelong.

6. **Reflexologists can tell me secrets and history about my life through my hands and feet and tell me the real reason of the health issues I am experiencing. This is something even my doctor can tell me.** A reflexologist is only a professional who helps you achieve the benefits of reflexology by offering you therapy sessions. While he or she may be able to detect your problem and heal it using the reflexology techniques, they cannot read out your life, history or secrets by touching or massaging your hands and feet. Don't even believe anyone who claims anything of that sort.

7. **One session is all I need to get all the positive energies and health benefits and I will experience it the moment I finish with my therapy.** Don't even expect to achieve all that reflexology has to offer you the moment you get up from the table. This is very unrealistic. While you will feel a lot of positive energy, relaxation and relief from pain after your very first therapy, just like any other form of treatment it requires that you stick to it and experience multiple sessions before you can actually claim the benefits.

In short, all these statements are wrong and should not be followed. Reflexology is not a narrow concept. It takes much more in treating a person with any condition than simply sticking to blank statements. So learn about it more and find out why all these statements are myths.

On the other hand, the reality about reflexology is that every human being is different. From age factor, to exposure to different environments to genetics, there is a conscious connection between an individual and reflexology which is unique. For professional reflexologists, it is very important to educate their clients so that they don't assume such things or simply follow the blank statements made by other people. Similarly, when you visit a reflexologist, make sure you ask them as many questions as you like to get rid of the confusions. Learn and educate yourself so that your mind opens and accepts reflexology as it is.

Reflexology Charts and Maps

So we will study the foot map and hand map separately here for better understanding. Professional reflexologist use pressure applied to reflex areas on the sole of the foot for the purpose of communicating with the corresponding organs and parts of the body through the central nervous system. This helps them in function at their best.

Foot Map

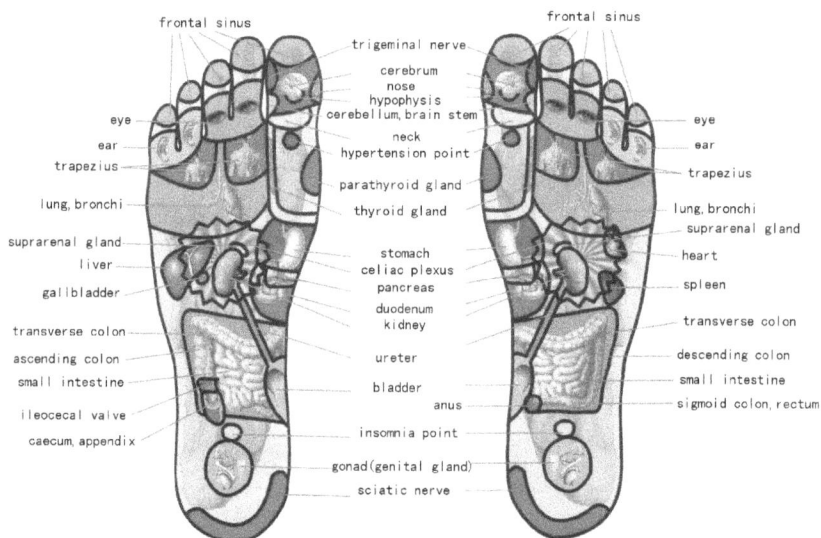

Your feet have reflex areas spread around corresponding with different organs in your body using the body's anatomy. This includes areas on your heels and toes, for instance, reflecting the lower back and head respectively.

The Right Sole

Your right foot map has reflex areas that correspond with the right side of your body. Similarly, the right arm reflex areas relates to the right arm. The reflex for liver on the right foot is much larger than the one highlighted on the right foot since most part of the liver falls on the right side of the body.

Left Sole

Your left foot corresponds with organs that fall on the left side of your body. The pancreas, stomach and the heart reflex sites on the left foot are significantly bigger than those on the right foot map since these organs are basically situation more towards the left side of the body.

Top Side Left Foot

The reflex areas on the top side of the left foot represent the left side of the body. To make it easy for yourself, know that the reflex area indicating spine falls on the inside area of the food and the shoulder reflex area is towards the outside.

The reflex areas for upper back, breast, chest, and lung are represented as one big area in the top center of your food. However, the lungs and chest reflex area lie in the same way behind the back of the foot as well.

Inside the Foot

The 'inside' view of the foot clearly displays the reflex area corresponding with the spine. This runs along the inside of the food. The big toe represents the neck, the area between the balls of the foot is the shoulder blades and the base of the heel is considered the tailbone of the spine.

The spine that runs inside the foot area includes the cervical, upper back, middle back, lower back and tail bone. Other than these, you will also see neck/brain stem, head/brain, face/sinus, teeth/gums/jaw, top of the shoulders, lungs/chest/breast/upper back, lower back, lymph glands, and uterus on this part of the foot.

Top of Right Foot

On top of the right foot, you will see reflex areas that address to the organs that fall on the right side of the body – such as the right leg and arm. There's a point highlighted on the right foot halfway down, which is known as the 'waistline'. The organs near the upper back area are mapped above this point. The internal organs and lower back are encased below. The groin and lymph gland reflex areas are wrapped near the ankle.

Outside Foot

The reflex areas that appear on top of the foot start with the shoulder area that runs across the toes and fingers. The side of the foot corresponds with the elbow and arm area of the body. Towards the ankle there are reflexes corresponding with reproductive organs. The curve around the ankle bone is reserved for the hip and sciatic nerve.

Hand Maps

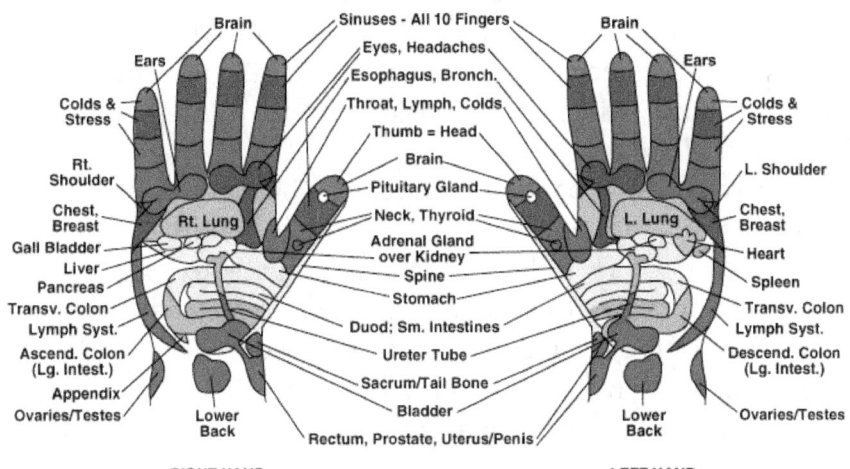

Just like the feet, the anatomy of your body is mapped on different reflex areas on the backs and fronts of your hands. The reflex area that corresponds with the head is located on the top of the thumbs and fingers. As far as the broken lines on the hands are concerned, this is where the reflex areas overlap.

Left Palm

Just like it was for the feet, the reflex areas on the left palm correspond to the left side of your body; starting with the neck and head areas on the top of the fingers and tailbone on the wrist. As far as the shoulder reflex is concerned, it is located towards the outside of the hand while the spine reflex is on the inside.

Right Palm

The right side of your body is mirrored on the reflex areas of your right palm. Your right hand is where the right side of your body corresponds to. Since there are different internal organs on the two sides of the body, there are differences between the reflexology maps for the left and right hands. For instance, the reflex area representing the lever will only fall on your right palm since the liver is on the right side of the body. The liver reflex will be totally missing from your left palm.

Top of Left Hand

There are a series of banded reflex areas that can be found on top of the left hand. This will directly correspond with the left side of your body including all the internal and external organs that are on our left. In addition to the internal organs, the top side of the left hand will also represent the left side of the body starting from the head to the knee. Reflex areas for fallopian tubes, lymph glands, and groin are present on the wrist.

Top of Right Hand

As mentioned earlier, the reflex areas on the right hand are linked with the internal and external organs of the right side of your body. The "waistline" is present at the base of the long bones. The reflex area for the upper back is located right above the waistline, while the hips, lower back and other internal organs they protect lie below the waistline reflex.

How to Use the Charts

You have finally reached to the most crucial part of the book – how to use the charts and apply reflexology in your life. It is ideal if you seek professional help to learn the exact technique of pressure application to make reflexology beneficial for you. However, here are step-by-step instructions how you can use the charts (details about the correspondence of body and internal organs with hands and feet) for your own benefits. Here's how you do it:

Sinuses/Brain/Head

The left side of your brain and head, as well as the left sinuses is corresponded with the segment of your left foot and left hand's fingers.
To apply the technique:
Foot – Use the technique of thumb-walk down to each toe on your left foot and make multiple passes. In case you are doing it yourself, use the same technique but thumb-walk up instead of down to the toes.
Hand – Use the technique of thumb-walking passes across fingers and thumb. For self-help, finger-walk across the fingers and thumb using your other hand.

Pituitary

The reflex area corresponding with the pituitary lies at the center of the big toe in the feet and the thumb in the hands. The left toe and left thumb will correspond to the left part of the pituitary gland.

Foot – Use the hook and back-up technique of reflexology on your big toe. In you want to do this yourself, apply the hook and backup technique using your index finger sliding it from the top.

Hand – Similarly, apply the same hook and backup techniques on the thumb of your left hand. If you are applying this reflexology technique by yourself, use your index finger for the application of pressure for hook and back-up technique.

Ear and Eye

The base of the toes of the foot and the base of the fingers on the hands are corresponded with the ear, inner ear and the eye. For instance, if you want to relief the left size of your ear, inner ear and left eye, you must apply the technique on your left foot and left hand.

Foot – To relieve the foot, hold the pad with one hand and apply the pressure on the base of the toes with other hand using the thumb-walk technique. In case you are doing it by yourself, apply a gentle pinch in between the webbings between toes.

Hands – Pinch the space between the fingers by gently apply the pressure there multiple times. For self-help reflexology technique, use your own other hand to gently apply pressure or pinch the webbings between your fingers.

Teeth and Face

The face and the teeth correspond with the reflex areas located at the bands that run across the tops of top of the thumb and all the fingers in your hands and on top of each toe on your foot. The left side of your face and teeth will correspond with the left food and hand and vice versa.

Foot – If someone else is doing it for you, use both the hands to apply pressure on the bands on top of teach toe using the thumb-walk technique. Make sure you make several passes in a single session. As a self-help technique, use one of your hands to make several thumb-walking passes across each toe.

Hands – Similarly, for hands apply the pressure using the same thumb-walk technique across the thumb and each finger. When doing it yourself, use your own hand to apply thumb-walking technique gently put pressure on the reflexes across the fingers and thumb.

Thyroid, Neck and Throat

The parathyroid and thyroid glands are corresponded on the reflex areas on the big toes on the feet and thumbs on the hand. On the other hand, throat and neck are represented on the digit and toe respectively.

Foot – With the help of thumb-walking pressure applying technique, work on the reflex areas right on the bands of your big toe. You will follow the same technique for self-help, however, make sure you make several passes for great benefits.

Hands – Again, in a series of passes, thumb-walk across the bands on the lower end of the thumb. When doing it yourself, use your other hand to apply the finger-walking technique in the same manner in a series of passes.

Upper Back, Lung and Chest

The upper palm side of the hand and the ball of the foot correspond with the upper back, lung and chest area of the body. If you want to treat the left side of your upper back, lung and chest, then apply reflexology technique to your left hand and left foot.

Foot – Thumb-walk each part of the ball of the foot. This is done in a series of passes and one of the hands holds the toes in place to apply the right pressure. To perform the self-help technique, place a foot-roller on the ground while you are seated or in the standing position. Place your left foot on the roller and roll over the ball with your foot. Make sure you apply a little pressure while rolling.

Hands – Hold the fingers in place with one hand and use the other hand to thumb-walk up the palm. Do multiple series. For self-help, apply the same thumb-walk up technique on your arm without holding the fingers. Again, do this by applying series of passes in a single reflexology session.

Shoulder

The right shoulder corresponds to a reflex area right under the smallest toe of the right foot and below the little finger on the left hand. So when addressing the right shoulder, focus on applying the reflexology techniques to your right hand and foot.

Foot – Use one hand to hold the toes back and with the other hand apply the thumb-walk technique up the shoulder area. For self-help, place your right foot on the roller and tilt your foot towards the little toe to apply pressure on that side. Roll the roller a few times to address the shoulder areas.

Hand – Hold the fingers with one hand while using the other one to thumb-walk up right below the little finger area. Make a series of several passes for great results. If you wish to do it yourself, simply apply the thumb –walk up technique to apply pressure on the area.

Heart

The foot ball right under the big toe on the foot and the palm area below the thumb corresponds with the heart. It is ideal to use your left foot and hand for this purpose since the heart predominantly lies on the left side of the body.
Foot – Hold the toes with one hand and using the other hand apply the thumb-walking technique up the foot. Apply several passes. For self help, you can still use your one hand to hold the toes and use your other hand to apply thumb-walk technique through the area in several passes.
Hand – Hold fingers back with one hand and with the other thumb-walk right below the left thumb reflex. If you want to do it yourself, use the finger-walking technique instead of the thumb-walk and apply pressure on the same area.

Gallbladder and Liver

To apply reflexology here, you will have to work on your right hand and right foot since the liver is primarily located on the right side of the body. Similarly, the gallbladder is also reflected only on the right hand and foot.
Foot – Hold the foot stead and keep your toes back with the help of your hand. With another hand, address the right reflex area on the foot and use the thumb-walk technique to apply pressure. To do it yourself, thumb walk the same area across the arch while keeping the toes back with your other hand.

Hands – Keeping your fingers at the back with your hand, thumb-walk across the palm in an upside down direction. Perform several passes. To do this reflexology technique by yourself, use a golf ball and roll it through the center of the palm with the help of other hand. Don't forget to apply gentle pressure while you perform this technique.

Stomach

The stomach as well as the spleen can be addressed by hitting the upper arch of the right foot and the center of the right palm.

Foot - Keep your foot steady and hold the toes with one hand. With another hand, apply thumb-walk technique for pressure in a cross direction moving towards the smallest toe. For self-help technique, apply the same technique with your own hands holding your toes tightly with one hand.

Hand – Apply thumb walking on in the downward direction on the center of the palm. Make sure you hold the fingers back while you apply pressure to the area. To do it yourself, again, use a golf ball and apply pressure on the reflexes as you roll it throughout the stomach and spleen reflexes.

Pancreas

For this reflexology session, you will once again have to use your left foot and left hand since the major part of the pancreas is positioned across the middle of arch on your left foot. Similarly, the heel of your hand can be addressed for the application of reflexology techniques to correspond to your pancreas.

Foot – With one hand hold the toes back and keep your foot steady. Apply the thumb-walking technique from bottom to top to apply the pressure. For self-help technique, thumb-walk as you keep your toes in your hand. This time, apply the pressure towards the little toe direction to be more effective.

Hand – Apply the thumb-walk down technique right under the thumb on your left hand. Make sure you hold your fingers during the reflexology session. On the other hand, use the gold ball if you wish to do it yourself. Hold a golf ball in your left hand and with the help your right hand, roll it and apply pressure throughout the area.

Kidney

If you wish to address the left kidney, then you must focus on your left food and hand and vice versa. The kidney is represented in the center of the foot. On the palm, it is located at the base of the webbing between the thumb and first finger.

Foot – Keep your toes stress and hold it with one hand as you perform this technique. Apply the pressure using the thumb-walking technique right in the center of your left foot. For self-help purpose, use the same technique to apply pressure and keep your toes tight and back with the help of your hands.

Hands – Once you are able to locate the right reflexes for the kidney on your palm, apply thumb-walking technique in the downward direction and apply several passes. For self-help technique, use the same technique but in the opposite direction. Again, don't forget to apply it in a series of passes.

Hip/Sciatic Nerve

In order to address the left hip and sciatic nerve, focus on the outside of your top left foot. For the hand, these organs are located on the outer wrist of the left hand below the smallest finger on the corner.

Foot – Keep your foot steady as one hand holds the top part of your toes. Using the finger-walking technique, address the right reflexes and apply pressure. For self-help, thumb-walk down towards your ankle, making several passes and applying gentle pressure for the reflexology session.

Hand – Use the multiple-finger-walking technique to apply pressure to the area. This will be addressing your left hip. Make sure the other hand is placed on top of your fingers covering 1/3 of them. If you wish to do this yourself, use the tips of your fingers to apply pressure on the reflexes on top of your hand. Press several times for effective results.

Arm/Elbow

As mentioned before, your left elbow and left arm will be represented by your left foot and left hand and vice versa. Thus, in order to address the left elbow and arm, pay attention to the upper portion of your outer foot right on the edge near the smallest toe. This will exactly be the same position on the arm but on the palm.

Foot – Keep your foot steady and your toes tight by placing the fingers of one hand on top of it. With another hand, thumb-walk on the edge of the foot in the upward direction. Make multiple passes. For self-help purpose, apply pressure on the same reflexes with your fingers using the finger-walking technique.

Hand – Keep your hand steady and hold your fingers with one hand. Apply pressure with both thumb and fingers as you gently pinch the edge of your hand. For self-help technique, do the same process with your thumb on your palm and fingers on top of the hand and gently pinch the fleshy outer edge of your hand.

Spine

The spine is very smartly divided between the right and left side of the body since it falls exactly in the center. This is exactly how it can be addressed using your hands and feet. The right half of your spine can be addressed on the inner edge of the right foot and the inner edge of the right hand.
Foot – Using the thumb-walking technique to apply pressure, gently press the edge of your foot in a series of passes. Make sure you apply gentle pressure. Also, don't forget to keep your foot stead and controlled with one hand. For self-help technique, Make several thumb walking passes with your own hand.
Hand – Keep your hands steady and hold your fingers tight and back with one hand. With the other hand, apply the pressure on the edge of the thumb towards the wrist in the upward direction using the thumb-walking technique. To do it yourself, hold your hand around the wrist and using the thumb-walking technique, apply pressure on the entire area effectively.
These are the most common and simple ways to use the charts. Relax your muscles, address your internal organs and treat them without getting detailed examinations and surgeries.

Reducing Stress with Reflexology – Real Techniques

In addition to using the techniques of reflexology for treatment, one of the ultimate goals people achieve using reflexology is to relax themselves. In fact, reflexology is a great way to create a relaxing experience when you need it the most. After all, it is the best way to prevent wear and tear on our system and de-stress ourselves from our tough routines. While we all are under some type or level of stress and it has become a part of our lives, continuous stress can lead to the development of various health issues.

The demands of our daily lives lead to various health problems that we experience regularly. Whether you suffer from migraines, insomnia, fatigue or digestive problems, the root of most of these health problems can be associated with the level of stress you experience. Stress is a major side effect of your own environmental, physical, emotional and lifestyle factors. Thus, it can be totally unavoidable sometimes.

In order to start your relaxation-from-reflexology therapy, create a very relaxing, soothing environment for yourself. You can do this to pamper yourself or you can help a loved one achieve inner peace and relaxation as you help him or her with the reflexology techniques.

Some great ideas before you get started with the session, start with:

1. Soft, lowered lights
2. Your favorite soft music (you can also use music they use for meditation and yoga)
3. Your favorite aroma
4. Some candles to simply lighten up your mood and make the place more calming and soothing.
5. A seating arrangement (maybe)

In case, you are doing it for someone else (maybe your significant other), make sure you arrange everything according to their preferences. Once you are done with the setting, the whole reflexology experience will take you to the next level altogether. It will not only make you or the other person comfortable, but will also help you achieve the ultimate goal of reflexology – i.e. de-stressing yourself!

Final Word

If you wish to get your reflexology sessions with a professional reflexologist in addition to, or instead of, self-application of reflexology techniques at home all by yourself, check the credentials of the practitioner for any membership or any qualification from different reflexology organizations. However, it is important to remember that the standards of reflexology have changed recently and thus it is very important to check with prospective practitioners about their professional experience as well as the date and duration of their qualification. The most reliable option would be one where reflexologists have at least completed a course comprising of 50 hours or more along with one year's experience. It is also important to bear in mind those practitioners who have expanded into other areas like offering other complementary therapies or selling products may not be very reliable as experienced reflexologist.

This book clearly highlights how you can carry out reflexology techniques yourself and address different parts of your body through the corresponding reflexes present on your hand and feet. Other than that, the information shared in this book will help you understand reflexology and help you differentiate between the facts and myths associated with the practice. In addition to this, the charts will help you understand the connection of all the organs in your body with your hands and feet. Last but not the least, the book also teaches how you can apply the technique of reflexology to get rid of pains, illnesses, and achieve your ultimate goal of relaxation.

Use the information shared in this book in your best interest and start applying reflexology in your life. Your hands and feet are the doorway to your entire body and by treating them right, you can successfully keep up with your health. You are just one step away from enjoying a better and much peaceful life. So get started now and experience the magical benefits of reflexology.

Best of luck!

www.ingramcontent.com/pod-product-compliance
Lightning Source LLC
Chambersburg PA
CBHW070841290526
45795CB00002B/942